EVERYTHING ABOUT BONE CANCER NUTRITION

A Comprehensive Guide To Dietary Strategies, Nutrient-Rich Foods, Supplements, Meal Plans For Effective Management And Improved Quality Of Life

WALTON USELTON

DISCLAIMER

The content in this book is based on the author's expertise and understanding of food and nutrition. The author is not linked or associated with any corporation, business, or person. This book is designed for informative purposes only and should not be interpreted as professional medical advice. Readers should get medical advice before making any changes to their diet or lifestyle. The author takes no responsibility or liability for any repercussions arising from the use of the information included in this book.

ABOUT THIS BOOK

"Bone Cancer Nutrition" is an essential resource that highlights the crucial role diet plays in controlling bone cancer. Its pages include a wealth of knowledge that not only informs but also empowers those confronting this difficult illness. At the center of This book is a thorough grasp of bone cancer, from its different forms to the intricate interaction of causes and risk factors. By unraveling the riddles of chronic conditions, readers find clarity and confidence in their path to better health.

This book's purpose is to explain the importance of critical nutrients for bone health. From calcium to vitamin D, each nutrient is thoroughly investigated to determine its significance in bone strength and resilience. This core understanding prepares readers for Chapter 2, which guides them through the process of creating a balanced diet suited to their unique requirements.

This book helps readers to confidently manage their nutritional intake by providing practical guidance on meal planning and portion management.

Furthermore, "Bone Cancer Nutrition" goes beyond dietary advice to explore the often-overlooked topic of hydration and its tremendous influence on bone health. By emphasizing the need for proper hydration and giving practical advice for remaining hydrated, this book equips readers with all of the skills they need to optimize their dietary routine.

As readers proceed through the chapters, they gain essential insights into foods that encourage bone health and those to avoid. From calcium-rich dairy products to the dangers of processed meats and sugary drinks, each tip is supported by evidence-based research, allowing readers to make more educated decisions.

Furthermore, this book goes beyond dietary recommendations to include weight control, symptom management, and the nuances of nutrition throughout therapy. Whether navigating surgery, chemotherapy, or radiation treatment, readers take comfort in the professional counsel provided in these pages.

This book's emphasis on long-term nutrition and survival, including switching to a post-treatment diet and continuing careful bone health monitoring, is also significant. By addressing survivors' comprehensive requirements, from mental health to access to resources and support networks, "Bone Cancer Nutrition" serves as a beacon of hope and guidance on the path to recovery and resilience.

INTRODUCTION

Understanding Bone Cancer

Bone cancer is an uncommon kind of cancer that originates in the bones. Unlike tumors that travel to the bones from other regions of the body, bone cancer develops inside the bone. This makes it different and, at times, more difficult to cure. However, with advances in medical science and a thorough approach to therapy, many people who have been diagnosed with bone cancer may still live productive lives.

What Is Bone Cancer?

Bone cancer is a disorder in which abnormal cells multiply uncontrolled inside bone tissue. These aberrant cells may become tumors, either benign (non-cancerous) or malignant (cancerous). Malignant bone tumors are classified as bone cancer.

Types Of Bone Cancer

There are various forms of bone cancer, each with unique features and treatment options. The most popular kinds are:

1. Osteosarcoma is the most common kind of bone cancer, mostly affecting the bones surrounding the knee, although it may grow in other bones.

2. Chondrosarcoma: This kind of bone cancer originates in cartilage cells and often affects the pelvis, legs, and arms.

3. Ewing sarcoma: Ewing sarcoma is more frequent in children and young people and affects the long bones of the body, such as the arms, legs, pelvis, and chest wall.

4. Chordomas often form near the base of the skull or in the bones of the spine.

Each kind of bone cancer may have a distinct treatment strategy, thus it is critical to correctly determine the type.

Causes And Risk Factors

The actual etiology of bone cancer is not yet completely known. However, some variables may raise your chance of getting bone cancer:

• Certain genetic disorders, including Li-Fraumeni syndrome and hereditary retinoblastoma, may raise the risk of bone cancer.

• Previous exposure to radiation treatment or atomic bombs may raise the chance of developing bone cancer.

• Paget's disease is a bone ailment that increases the likelihood of developing osteosarcoma.

• Certain forms of bone cancer are more prevalent in various age groups, while it may develop at any age.

Ewing sarcoma, for example, is typically seen in children and young adults.

Importance Of Diet In Bone Cancer Treatment

Nutrition is very important in the treatment of bone cancer. A well-balanced diet may improve general health while also strengthening the body's capacity to fight cancer and tolerate therapy. A proper diet may also help control symptoms and side effects of bone cancer and therapy, such as tiredness, nausea, and weight loss.

Overview Of This Book's Contents

In this book, we will look at the complex interaction between diet and bone cancer care. We will investigate how different nutrition and dietary regimens might improve treatment results and quality of life for people with bone cancer.

This book seeks to offer comprehensive counsel for patients, carers, and healthcare professionals, covering everything from the significance of certain nutrients in bone health to practical recommendations for maintaining a balanced diet throughout treatment. Whether you're looking for information on dietary supplements, meal planning, or dealing with side effects, this book will be a great resource on your path to better health and well-being.

CHAPTER ONE

Essential Nutrients for Bone Health

Calcium: Building Blocks Of Strong Bones

Calcium is often regarded as the most important vitamin for bone health and with good reason. It functions similarly to a building's cornerstone, providing the structural underpinning for bone density and strength. Consuming a proper quantity of calcium is critical, particularly throughout infancy and adolescence when bones are still growing. But don't worry, adults also need it to preserve bone density and avoid diseases like osteoporosis.

So, where do you acquire your daily calcium? Dairy items such as milk, cheese, and yogurt are great sources. However, if you are lactose intolerant or practice a plant-based diet, don't worry! Calcium may still be found in fortified plant-based milk substitutes, leafy greens like kale and broccoli, tofu, walnuts, and tinned fish like sardines and salmon (with bones).

Vitamin D, The Sunshine Vitamin

Vitamin D is important for bone health because it allows the body to absorb calcium more effectively. It's as if the sunshine ignites the calcium's ability to strengthen your bones. However, many individuals do not receive enough vitamin D, particularly those who live in places with little sunshine or spend the majority of their time inside.

To increase your vitamin D levels, spend time in the sun sensibly (approximately 10-30 minutes a few times each week). But don't forget the sunscreen! Additionally, include vitamin D-rich foods in your diet, such as fatty fish like salmon, tuna, and mackerel, egg yolks, fortified foods like orange juice and cereals, and UV-exposed mushrooms.

Phosphorus: Partner In Bone Formation

Phosphorus may not get as much attention as calcium and vitamin D, but it is as important for bone health. Consider it the dependable companion of calcium, working together to develop and preserve bone strength. Phosphorus is plentiful in protein-rich foods such as meat, poultry, fish, dairy products, nuts, seeds, and whole grains.

Ensuring a sufficient phosphorus intake is critical for good bone mineralization and overall bone health. Fortunately, most individuals may easily satisfy their phosphorus requirements with a well-balanced diet, without the need for extra supplements.

Magnesium Regulates Bone Health

Magnesium functions as a behind-the-scenes director, coordinating different processes in the body, including bone metabolism. It regulates calcium levels in the blood and aids in the structural development of bone structure. Calcium may not be used efficiently if magnesium levels are low, which might contribute to bone health difficulties.

Magnesium may be found in a wide range of foods, including leafy greens, nuts & seeds, whole grains, beans, lentils, and even dark chocolate. By integrating these items into your diet, you can ensure that you obtain an adequate dose of magnesium to promote bone health.

Vitamin K Strengthens Bone Density

Vitamin K is not as well-known as some of its equivalents, but it plays an important function in bone health by assisting in the production of proteins required for bone mineralization. It's like the reinforcement that keeps your bones strong and tough.

Leafy green foods such as kale, spinach, and collard greens are rich in vitamin K. Other vegetables that include it include broccoli, Brussels sprouts, and asparagus, as well as certain oils such as soybean and canola oil.

Calcium, vitamin D, phosphorus, magnesium, and vitamin K are vital elements that serve as the foundation for strong, healthy bones. By including a range of nutrient-dense foods in your diet, you can guarantee that your bones get the support they need to flourish throughout your life. So, whether it's a glass of milk, a plate of leafy greens, or a portion of salmon, remember that each mouthful contributes to your bone health journey.

CHAPTER TWO

Building A Balanced Diet

Importance Of A Balanced Diet

A well-balanced diet is essential for everyone, but especially for individuals facing bone cancer. A well-balanced diet supplies the nutrients needed to maintain general health and vigor, which is critical for dealing with the difficulties of cancer therapy. Protein, vitamins, minerals, and antioxidants are essential nutrients for immune system support, healing, and energy maintenance.

A well-balanced diet may also help manage the negative effects of cancer therapies such as chemotherapy and radiation therapy. For example, eating antioxidant-rich foods may help minimize inflammation and oxidative stress, whilst getting adequate protein boosts muscular strength and recovery. Furthermore, a well-balanced diet may help you maintain a healthy weight, which is essential for general health throughout cancer treatment.

Make A Meal Plan

Creating a meal plan may help you maintain a healthy diet, particularly during difficult times like cancer treatment. Begin by meeting with a trained dietician, who may create a meal plan tailored to your unique requirements and tastes. A meal plan usually contains a range of meals from various food categories to ensure optimal nutritional intake.

When creating a meal plan, include a variety of entire grains, lean meats, healthy fats, fruits, and vegetables. Aim for colorful fruits and vegetables, which are high in vitamins, minerals, and antioxidants. Whole grains give fiber and energy, whilst lean proteins like chicken, fish, tofu, and lentils promote muscle health and repair.

Incorporating Fruits And Vegetables

Fruits and vegetables are key components of a healthy diet, providing a variety of vitamins, minerals, and phytonutrients. To guarantee nutritional diversity, include a range of colors and varieties within your diet. Dark leafy greens, such as spinach and kale, are high in calcium and vitamin K, which are beneficial to bone health.

Incorporating fruits and veggies into your meals may be simple and enjoyable. Try mixing berries into your morning cereal or yogurt, munching on carrot sticks with hummus, or serving a colorful salad with lunch and supper. Consider combining fruits and veggies into smoothies for a handy and nutritious snack.

Choosing Lean Proteins

Protein is necessary for maintaining muscular strength, immunological function, and healing after cancer therapy.

Choose lean proteins to reduce your saturated fat consumption. Good choices include chicken, fish, eggs, tofu, tempeh, and legumes like beans and lentils.

Include lean proteins in your meals and snacks throughout the day to maintain optimal consumption. For example, include grilled chicken breast or fish into your main meals, add beans or lentils to soups and salads, and snack on Greek yogurt or cottage cheese for protein.

Managing Portion Sizes

Managing portion sizes is essential for a healthy diet and weight management during cancer treatment. While appropriate food intake is essential, overeating may contribute to weight gain.

Visual signals and portion control tactics may help you regulate portion amounts. For example, strive to fill half of your plate with fruits and vegetables, a quarter with lean protein, and the other quarter with nutritious grains or starchy veggies. Additionally, pay attention to your body's hunger and fullness signals, eating until you're satisfied but not excessively full.

While facing bone cancer, you may improve your general health and well-being by eating a balanced diet that includes fruits and vegetables, lean meats, and portion control. Working with a licensed dietitian may offer you personalized advice and support as you manage dietary issues and optimize your nutrition throughout treatment.

CHAPTER THREE

Hydration And Bone Health

Importance Of Hydration

Hydration is essential for general health and contributes significantly to bone health. Our bodies are around 60% water, and every cell, tissue, and organ needs enough hydration to operate properly. Hydration is critical for bone health because it helps to preserve bone integrity and strength.

Water plays an important role in many bodily functions, including nutrition delivery, waste removal, and temperature control. In terms of bone health, appropriate hydration ensures that vital minerals, such as calcium and magnesium, are delivered to the bones and contribute to their density and strength.

Bones may deteriorate due to a lack of water, leaving them more prone to fractures and other ailments.

Dehydration may also cause reduced joint lubrication, exacerbating illnesses such as arthritis and discomfort. As a result, keeping optimal water levels is critical for maintaining bone health and general wellness.

Recommended Daily Water Intake

The recommended daily water consumption varies by age, gender, activity intensity, and climate. However, a general recommendation for people is to drink at least 8-10 glasses of water every day. This translates to around 2-3 liters of water every day.

Individual water demands vary, and some conditions, such as strenuous activity or hot weather, may raise the body's fluid requirements. Paying attention to thirst signals and urine color may also assist in determining hydration levels. Clear or light-colored urine is usually indicative of appropriate hydration, however, dark urine may suggest dehydration.

Effects Of Dehydration On Bone Health

Dehydration may hurt bone health. When the body does not have enough water, it prioritizes the transfer of remaining fluids to key organs, frequently at the cost of less crucial tissues like bones. As a consequence, bones may become depleted of essential minerals, resulting in lower bone density and an increased risk of fractures.

Chronic dehydration may also damage the body's capacity to absorb calcium, a mineral necessary for bone strength. Without an appropriate amount of calcium, bones may weaken and fracture over time, increasing the risk of osteoporosis and other bone-related disorders.

Furthermore, dehydration may aggravate pre-existing bone and joint problems, such as arthritis, by decreasing joint lubrication and increasing bone friction. This may cause pain, stiffness, and reduced movement, affecting overall bone health.

Hydrating Foods And Beverages

In addition to drinking water, ingesting hydrating foods and drinks may aid in maintaining optimal hydration levels and bone health. Fruits and vegetables, which contain a lot of water, are great options for keeping hydrated. Cucumbers, watermelon, strawberries, oranges, celery, and lettuce are among the examples.

Additionally, some beverages, such as herbal teas, coconut water, and electrolyte-rich sports drinks, may help with hydration while also supplying critical nutrients. However, sugary and caffeinated drinks should be drunk in moderation since they might have a diuretic impact and possibly contribute to dehydration.

Tips To Stay Hydrated

Staying hydrated throughout the day is critical for bone health and general wellness. Here are some practical suggestions for staying well-hydrated:

1. Carry a reusable water bottle with you wherever you go to provide quick access to fluids throughout the day.

2. Set reminders on your phone or computer to drink water regularly, particularly if you are prone to forgetting.

3. To increase hydration, drink a glass of water when you wake up and before each meal.

4. Choose hydrating snacks, such as fresh fruits and vegetables, to increase your water consumption.

5. Limit your use of dehydrating liquids such as alcohol and caffeine, particularly in hot weather or during strenuous physical exercise.

6. Monitor your urine color to determine your hydration level; light yellow or clear pee indicates enough hydration.

7. Be aware of indicators of dehydration, such as thirst, dry mouth, weariness, and dizziness, and respond quickly by drinking water.

By adopting these techniques into your daily routine and prioritizing water, you may promote good bone health and general well-being. Remember that being hydrated is critical not just for bone health, but also for overall body function and vigor.

CHAPTER FOUR

Foods To Include In Your Diet

Dairy Products

Dairy products are an important part of a bone cancer patient's diet because they contain high levels of calcium, which is essential for bone health. When fighting bone cancer, keeping healthy bones is critical, and calcium plays an important part in this process. Dairy products including milk, yogurt, and cheese are high in calcium.

However, it is critical to choose low-fat or fat-free dairy products to reduce saturated fat consumption, which may be harmful to general health, particularly for those undergoing cancer treatment. Including dairy products in meals and snacks may be as easy as drinking a glass of milk in the morning, adding yogurt to smoothies or snacks, or putting cheese into salads or sandwiches.

Furthermore, for people who are lactose intolerant or prefer non-dairy choices, there are several fortified plant-based milk substitutes available that give comparable calcium benefits.

Leafy Greens

Leafy greens are nutritional powerhouses that should be included in the diets of everyone fighting bone cancer. These plants, such as spinach, kale, collard greens, and Swiss chard, are high in vitamins, minerals, and antioxidants, which promote general health and bone health.

One of the important elements present in leafy greens is vitamin K, which is essential for bone metabolism and helps regulate calcium levels in the body. Furthermore, leafy greens are high in calcium, magnesium, and other critical vitamins and minerals that improve bone health and density.

Leafy greens may be included in a variety of dishes, including salads, soups, stir-fries, and smoothies. They may also be steamed, sautéed, or baked as a side dish or combined with main entrees. Include a mix of leafy greens in your diet to ensure you obtain a wide range of nutrients to promote bone health.

Fish With Bones

Fish with edible bones, such as canned salmon or sardines, are ideal complements to a bone cancer patient's diet. These fish have high levels of calcium and vitamin D, both of which are necessary for bone health.

Calcium from fish bones is easily absorbed by the body, making it a good supply of this vital mineral. Furthermore, vitamin D aids in calcium absorption and helps regulate calcium levels in the body, resulting in strong and healthy bones.

Adding canned salmon or sardines to salads, sandwiches, or pasta dishes is an easy way to include bone-in fish into meals. These fish may also be mashed and spread on crackers or toast as a healthful snack. To gain the advantages of calcium and vitamin D, add bone-in fish to your diet regularly.

Nuts And Seeds

Nuts and seeds are nutrient-dense foods that may help bone cancer sufferers because they include high levels of calcium, magnesium, phosphorus, and other vital elements that promote bone health.

Almonds, sesame seeds, chia seeds, and sunflower seeds are especially high in calcium, making them ideal for a bone-healthy diet. Furthermore, nuts and seeds are high in healthy fats, protein, and fiber, which may give long-term energy and support general well-being throughout cancer treatment.

Adding nuts and seeds to your diet may be as easy as sprinkling them over salads, yogurt, or muesli, or eating them as a snack on their own. Nut butter, such as almond butter or tahini (produced from sesame seeds), may be spread over toast or used as a dip for fruits and vegetables.

Fortified Foods

Fortified foods are those that have been supplemented with extra nutrients, such as calcium and vitamin D, to increase their nutritional value. For bone cancer patients, integrating fortified foods into their diet will help them get more of these key bone-building minerals.

Orange juice, cereal, plant-based milk replacements, and tofu are all examples of fortified foods. These products may be a simple and accessible source of calcium and vitamin D, particularly for people who have dietary limitations or preferences that limit their use of conventional dairy products or fish with bones.

When choosing fortified foods, read the nutrition labels to ensure they contain enough quantities of calcium and vitamin D. Incorporate a variety of fortified foods into your diet to ensure you're receiving a wide range of nutrients to promote bone health throughout cancer treatment.

CHAPTER FIVE

Foods To Limit Or Avoid

Processed Meats

One of the most important concerns in a bone cancer diet is to avoid processed meats. These are meats that have been preserved using a variety of processes, including smoking, curing, and salting. While they may be handy and delicious, they often include a host of chemicals and preservatives that may be harmful to your health, particularly if you are facing cancer.

One of the primary issues of processed meats is their high salt level. Excessive salt consumption may cause water retention and aggravate swelling and pain, especially if you have bone cancer. Furthermore, many processed meats include nitrites and nitrates, substances related to an increased risk of cancer.

Furthermore, processed meats are generally heavy in harmful lipids, such as saturated and trans fats. These fats may cause inflammation in the body, which you should avoid while fighting cancer. Instead, include lean protein sources in your diet, such as chicken, fish, tofu, beans, and lentils.

Sugary Drinks

Sugary drinks are another food group that should be limited or avoided while controlling bone cancer. These include sodas, sugar-laden fruit juices, energy drinks, and sweetened teas. While these drinks may be pleasant, they are high in empty calories and may trigger blood sugar surges, which is not good for cancer patients.

Excess sugar intake has been related to obesity, inflammation, and insulin resistance, all of which may have a severe influence on your general health and well-being, particularly if you are facing a serious disease such as cancer. Instead of sugary drinks, choose water, herbal teas, or freshly squeezed juices with no added sugars. These solutions will help you stay hydrated without the negative effects of additional sugars.

High-Sodium Foods

Foods high in salt should be minimized or avoided in a bone cancer diet. Sodium is a mineral that is necessary for many body activities, but an excess of it may cause high blood pressure, fluid retention, and other health problems. Excessive salt consumption may aggravate edema and pain in people with bone cancer, so limit your sodium intake.

Processed foods are often the leading cause of elevated salt levels in the diet. These include canned soups, frozen meals, pre-packaged snacks, and fast food. To limit your sodium consumption, eat fresh, complete foods wherever feasible and prepare meals at home using herbs, spices, and other flavorings instead of salt.

Excess Alcohol

Limiting or avoiding excessive alcohol intake is also recommended for those with bone cancer. While moderate alcohol intake may not be harmful to everyone, excessive drinking may weaken the immune system, interact with medicines, and raise the chance of developing certain malignancies, including bone cancer.

Alcohol may also dehydrate the body, which is especially problematic for cancer patients who are already at risk of dehydration owing to treatment side effects or other causes. If you decide to consume alcohol, do it in moderation and remain hydrated by drinking lots of water.

Caffeine

Finally, while treating bone cancer, coffee should be used in moderation. While moderate caffeine consumption is generally regarded as safe for the majority of people, excessive caffeine consumption can cause dehydration, disrupt sleep, and exacerbate anxiety, all of which can hurt your overall health and well-being, particularly when dealing with a serious illness such as cancer.

Caffeine may be found in a variety of forms, including coffee, tea, energy drinks, and chocolate. If you prefer caffeinated drinks, consume them in moderation and be aware of how caffeine affects your body. If you notice that caffeine exacerbates any symptoms or adverse effects related to bone cancer therapy, consider switching to decaffeinated or herbal teas.

CHAPTER SIX

Maintaining A Healthy Weight

Importance Of Weight Management

Maintaining a healthy weight is critical for people with bone cancer. Proper weight control may improve overall health and quality of life. Weight control is important for bone cancer patients because it helps the body fight the illness and tolerate therapy.

Excess weight may put pressure on the bones and joints, increasing cancer's already uncomfortable symptoms. Being underweight, on the other hand, may weaken the body, making it more vulnerable to infections and limiting the energy required for treatment and recovery. As a result, reaching and maintaining an ideal weight is critical for successful bone cancer management.

Balance Calorie Intake And Expenditure

The fundamental principle of weight control is to balance calorie intake and expenditure. This balance is particularly important for bone cancer patients, whose bodies go through strenuous therapy and repair procedures. Calorie requirements vary according to age, gender, weight, height, exercise level, and stage of cancer.

To maintain a healthy weight, eat a well-balanced diet that includes all of the required nutrients while being aware of portion sizes. This contains an abundance of fruits, vegetables, lean meats, whole grains, and healthy fats. Monitoring calorie consumption may be beneficial, but it's also critical to ensure that the calories taken are nutrient-dense and promote general health.

Strategies For Weight Loss Or Gain

Depending on their specific circumstances, bone cancer patients may need to concentrate on either weight reduction or weight growth. For people who are overweight, progressive and sustained weight reduction may reduce stress on the bones and joints, increase mobility, and improve general well-being. This often entails producing a calorie deficit via a combination of dietary adjustments and increased physical activity.

Underweight individuals, on the other hand, may benefit from gaining weight to strengthen their bodies and enhance their capacity to endure therapy. This usually entails ingesting more calories than you burn, with a focus on nutrient-dense meals that encourage healthy weight gain. Working with a healthcare physician or certified dietitian may aid in the development of personalized weight-loss methods that are both safe and successful.

Incorporating Physical Activity

Physical exercise is an important part of weight control for bone cancer patients. While it may seem difficult, particularly during treatment, being active may provide various advantages, including increased strength, mobility, mood, and overall quality of life. Depending on one's ability and choices, activities might vary from simple workouts like walking, yoga, or swimming to more moderate or rigorous ones.

It is important to listen to your body and modify the intensity and duration of physical exercise appropriately. Starting gently and gradually increasing exercise levels may assist avoid weariness and reduce the chance of injury. Additionally, including strength training routines may help preserve muscle mass and bone density, which is very crucial for cancer patients.

Monitoring Progress

Monitoring progress is critical for effective weight control in individuals with bone cancer. Weight, food consumption, physical activity, and general well-being may all be tracked regularly to provide insight into what works and what needs to be changed. Keeping a food journal, utilizing mobile apps to monitor activity, and arranging frequent check-ins with healthcare professionals or dietitians may help you remain on track and make changes as required. Celebrating minor triumphs along the road may give inspiration and encouragement to keep working towards a healthy weight and a better quality of life.

CHAPTER SEVEN

Addressing Symptoms And Side Effects

Nausea And Vomiting

People getting treatment for bone cancer often feel nausea and vomiting. These symptoms may be upsetting and reduce a person's quality of life. However, there are techniques for dealing with them successfully.

Dietary changes may help relieve nausea and vomiting. It is critical to concentrate on eating bland, readily digested meals that are easy on the stomach. This includes crackers, bread, bananas, rice, and applesauce. Avoiding oily, spicy, or too-rich meals might also assist in alleviating these symptoms.

In addition to dietary adjustments, keeping hydrated is essential. Drinking clear fluids throughout the day, such as water, herbal teas, or ginger ale, will calm the stomach and keep you hydrated. It is important to avoid sugary or caffeinated drinks since they might exacerbate nausea.

Furthermore, including ginger in your diet may alleviate nausea. Ginger has natural anti-nausea effects and may be ingested in a variety of ways, including ginger tea, ginger sweets, and adding raw ginger to meals.

If nausea and vomiting continue after dietary changes, your doctor may prescribe medicines. Antiemetics and other drugs that inhibit the nausea response may give substantial relief. It is important to follow your healthcare provider's instructions for drug dose and timing.

Loss Of Appetite

Another typical symptom associated with bone cancer is loss of appetite. When your hunger is low, it's critical to concentrate on nutrient-dense meals to guarantee enough nutrition.

One technique for combating appetite loss is to eat small, regular meals throughout the day instead of big ones. This may help to reduce overpowering sensations of fullness and make eating more bearable. Additionally, including high-calorie, protein-rich foods in meals and snacks might help increase calorie consumption.

It's also important to pay attention to your body's hunger signals and eat when you're hungry, even if it's outside of regular meal hours. Keeping a range of nutritious snacks on hand, such as nuts, cheese, yogurt, or fruit, might help you fulfill your cravings when they arise.

If cooking becomes difficult owing to weariness or other symptoms, try asking the assistance of friends or family members, or look into handy meal choices like pre-made meals or meal delivery services.

Fatigue

Fatigue is a common complaint among those being treated for bone cancer. While it may seem daunting, there are ways to manage tiredness and conserve energy throughout the day.

One strategy is to prioritize activities and save energy for important tasks. This might include outsourcing non-essential duties to others or breaking down bigger jobs into smaller, more manageable ones. Planning relaxation breaks during the day might also assist in avoiding overexertion.

In addition to pacing oneself, a well-balanced diet is vital for overcoming weariness. Consuming a range of nutrient-dense meals, such as fruits, vegetables, lean meats, and whole grains, helps give consistent energy throughout the day. It's also important to remain hydrated by consuming lots of water.

Gentle exercise may also assist with weariness. Walking, swimming, and yoga are all activities that might help you feel more energized and less tired. However, you must listen to your body and prevent overexertion.

If weariness remains after these methods, you must contact your healthcare staff. They may assist in determining the underlying reasons for weariness and prescribe further measures, such as drugs or supportive therapy.

Changes In Taste And Odor

Changes in taste and smell are frequent side effects of bone cancer therapy, and they may have a substantial influence on appetite and nutrition.

Understanding how to handle these changes may aid in ensuring proper nutrition throughout therapy.

One way to cope with changes in taste and scent is to explore various flavors and textures to discover meals that appeal to you. This might include testing new recipes or using herbs and spices to improve the flavor of dishes.

Furthermore, concentrating on foods with strong flavors, such as citrus fruits, garlic, or spicy dishes, may assist in exciting the taste buds and improve meal quality. Marinating meats and vegetables in tasty sauces or dressings may also assist in disguising disagreeable flavors.

It is critical to be patient and adaptable with your nutritional choices during this period. What were your favorite meals before therapy may no longer be appealing, and that's OK. Trying new foods and flavors may help you broaden your culinary horizons and make meals more pleasurable.

Digestive Issues

Constipation, diarrhea, and stomach pain are all possible side effects of bone cancer therapy. These symptoms may be distracting and unpleasant, but they can usually be treated with dietary and lifestyle adjustments.

Increasing fiber intake is one way to address digestive disorders like constipation. Fiber-rich meals, such as fruits, vegetables, whole grains, and legumes, may aid with regular bowel movements. To avoid worsening symptoms, gradually increase your fiber intake and stay hydrated.

For those suffering from diarrhea, avoiding meals and drinks that might aggravate symptoms, such as spicy foods, coffee, and high-fat foods, may help. Instead, eat bland, readily digested items like rice, bananas, and bread.

Incorporating probiotic-rich foods into your diet, such as yogurt, kefir, or sauerkraut, may also support a healthy balance of gut flora and aid with digestive disorders.

If your digestive problems continue or worsen, you should see your doctor. They may assist in identifying underlying causes and recommending suitable therapies or actions for optimal symptom management.

CHAPTER EIGHT

Nutrition During Treatment

Surgery

Surgery is a frequent therapy for bone cancer, especially if the tumor is localized and has not progressed to other regions of the body. The purpose of surgery is to remove as much malignant tissue as possible while maintaining function in the afflicted limb or region. Proper nutrition before and after surgery is critical for the healing process and overall result.

Before surgery, it is essential to eat a well-balanced diet that contains enough protein, vitamins, and minerals. Protein is essential for tissue repair and immunological function, so consume lean meats, fish, eggs, dairy, legumes, and nuts. Vitamins and minerals including vitamin C, vitamin D, calcium, and zinc are also beneficial to bone health and wound healing. Include lots of fruits, veggies, whole grains, and dairy products in your diet to ensure you obtain enough nutrients.

Following surgery, your body needs additional nutrients to aid in healing and rehabilitation. Depending on the degree of the operation, you may have a diminished appetite or trouble eating, so concentrate on nutrient-dense meals. Consume modest, regular meals and snacks throughout the day to satisfy your energy and nutritional requirements. Include protein-rich meals such as chicken, turkey, fish, tofu, beans, and dairy products to aid in tissue regeneration and recuperation. Staying hydrated is also crucial, so consume lots of fluids like water, herbal teas, and diluted fruit juices.

Chemotherapy

Chemotherapy is a systemic treatment that employs chemicals to eliminate cancer cells throughout the body. While chemotherapy may be useful in treating bone cancer, it can also have adverse consequences on your nutritional condition and general well-being. Managing these side effects with a good diet is critical during chemotherapy treatment.

Chemotherapy often causes nausea and vomiting, making it difficult to consume and maintain sufficient nutrition. To ease these symptoms, eat bland, easily digestible meals such as crackers, bread, rice, bananas, and clear broth. Avoid oily, spicy, or strong-smelling meals, since these might cause nausea.

Chemotherapy may also cause changes in taste and appetite, making certain meals less appetizing. Experiment with various flavors and textures to identify meals that appeal to you.

Adding herbs, spices, and marinades to your dishes may assist to improve flavor and make them more pleasurable.

Furthermore, chemotherapy might weaken the immune system, raising the risk of infection. To boost your immune system throughout chemotherapy, eat a nutrient-dense diet rich in fruits, vegetables, whole grains, lean meats, and healthy fats. These foods include critical vitamins, minerals, and antioxidants that boost the immune system and improve general health.

Radiation Therapy

Radiation treatment employs high-energy radiation to destroy cancer cells and reduce tumors. While radiation therapy is a localized treatment that focuses on certain regions of the body, it may nevertheless have an impact on your nutrition and general well-being.

Proper diet is vital during radiation therapy to help your body deal with the effects of the treatment and promote recovery.

Fatigue is a typical side effect of radiation treatment, making it difficult to maintain a good diet and exercise routine. To prevent weariness, choose nutrient-dense meals that give long-lasting energy, such as whole grains, lean meats, fruits, and vegetables. Eating small, regular meals and snacks throughout the day might also assist in maintaining your energy levels.

Radiation therapy may also cause skin irritation and inflammation in the treatment region. To calm sensitive skin and encourage healing, consume foods high in vitamins A and C, zinc, and antioxidants. Include carrots, sweet potatoes, citrus fruits, berries, nuts, and seeds in your diet to promote skin health and wound healing.

Radiation treatment may also induce changes in appetite and taste, comparable to chemotherapy. Experiment with various cuisines and flavors to see what suits you best, and don't be hesitant to try new dishes or ingredients. It's also crucial to keep hydrated by consuming lots of fluids including water, herbal teas, and electrolyte-rich drinks, which help flush out toxins and improve general health.

Targeted Therapy

Targeted therapy is a method of treatment that uses medicines or other substances to detect and destroy particular cancer cells while causing little harm to healthy cells. Unlike chemotherapy, which affects all rapidly dividing cells in the body, targeted treatment focuses on cancer cells based on genetic abnormalities or other distinguishing traits.

A proper diet during targeted therapy is critical for supporting the body's response to treatment and minimizing adverse effects. Focus on a well-balanced diet rich in fruits, vegetables, whole grains, lean meats, and healthy fats to offer critical nutrients and promote overall health.

Gastrointestinal difficulties such as diarrhea, constipation, or nausea are one possible adverse effect of targeted treatment. To assist with these symptoms, eat fiber-rich foods like fruits, vegetables, whole grains, and legumes, which may regulate digestion and improve bowel regularity. Stay hydrated by drinking lots of fluids. Avoid coffee and alcohol, which may irritate the digestive system.

Another negative effect of targeted treatment is weariness, which may make it difficult to maintain a balanced diet and keep active. To prevent weariness, choose nutrient-dense meals that give long-lasting energy, such as lean proteins, complex carbs, and healthy fats.

Eating small, regular meals and snacks throughout the day might also assist in maintaining your energy levels.

Furthermore, targeted treatment may alter the taste and fragrance of food, making certain meals less desirable. Experiment with various flavors and textures until you discover things that you like, and don't be hesitant to try new recipes or ingredients. It's also critical to keep hydrated by consuming enough of fluids including water, herbal teas, and electrolyte-rich drinks to promote general health and well-being.

Immunotherapy

Immunotherapy is a treatment that employs the body's immune system to combat cancer. Unlike chemotherapy, which directly targets cancer cells, immunotherapy enhances the immune system's capacity to recognize and eliminate cancer cells. Proper diet during immunotherapy is critical for supporting the body's immune response and improving treatment results.

Inflammation is a possible adverse effect of immunotherapy that may affect many regions of the body, including the digestive system. Anti-inflammatory foods including fruits, vegetables, whole grains, fatty fish, nuts, and seeds may help decrease inflammation and improve gastrointestinal health. Avoid processed meals, sugary snacks, and fried foods, since they may all lead to inflammation.

Another complication of immunotherapy is exhaustion, which may make it difficult to maintain a good diet and keep active. To prevent weariness, choose nutrient-dense meals that give long-lasting energy, such as lean proteins, complex carbs, and healthy fats. Eating small, regular meals and snacks throughout the day might also assist in maintaining your energy levels.

Furthermore, immunotherapy might reduce appetite and alter taste and scent, making some meals less desirable. Experiment with various flavors and textures until you discover things that you like, and don't be hesitant to try new recipes or ingredients. It's also critical to keep hydrated by consuming enough of fluids including water, herbal teas, and electrolyte-rich drinks to promote general health and well-being.

CHAPTER NINE

Nutritional Support And Supplements

Importance Of Nutritional Support

Nutritional assistance is critical for those with bone cancer because it improves general health, manages symptoms, and supports treatment success. When dealing with bone cancer, the body's nutritional requirements often vary as a result of increased metabolic demands, medication side effects, and the disease's influence on appetite and digestion.

One of the key objectives of nutritional support is to ensure that patients obtain enough nutrients to preserve their strength, energy levels, and immunological function. Adequate diet may also help manage common side symptoms including tiredness, nausea, and weight loss in cancer patients.

Furthermore, an appropriate diet may improve the body's capacity to tolerate treatment options such as chemotherapy, radiation therapy, and surgery. Nutritional assistance may help bone cancer patients achieve better treatment results and a higher quality of life by supplying the required nutrients.

Choosing Supplements Carefully

When contemplating supplements for bone cancer patients, it is critical to pick intelligently and proceed with caution. While supplements may occasionally augment traditional therapy and ease specific symptoms, they should not be used as a substitute for a healthy diet or prescription pharmaceuticals.

Before adding any supplements to a treatment plan, speak with a healthcare expert, ideally one who specializes in cancer care and nutrition. A healthcare expert may evaluate an individual's requirements, possible interactions with drugs or therapies, and the general safety and effectiveness of certain supplements.

When choosing supplements, prioritize those that treat documented nutritional deficits or alleviate particular symptoms or adverse effects. Calcium and vitamin D supplements, for example, may be prescribed to preserve bone health, whilst omega-3 fatty acids may aid in inflammation reduction and heart health.

Risks And Benefits Of Supplementation

Making educated judgments requires a thorough understanding of the dangers and benefits of supplements. While certain supplements may provide advantages such as immunological support, symptom alleviation, or better nutritional status, they may also be harmful, especially when taken incorrectly or in large dosages.

Some supplements may interfere with drugs or therapies, lowering their efficacy or producing side effects. Others may have inadequate scientific evidence to support their use in cancer treatment, or they may worsen certain symptoms or diseases.

To balance the possible advantages and hazards of supplementing, healthcare practitioners must carefully examine and monitor the situation on an ongoing basis. Regular contact with a healthcare team may assist ensure that supplements are utilized safely and successfully as part of a multifaceted treatment strategy.

Herbal Remedies

Individuals looking for alternative or complementary cancer therapy often seek herbal therapies, such as plant extracts and traditional medications. While some herbs may offer anecdotal evidence that they might help manage cancer symptoms or improve quality of life, their safety and effectiveness are unknown.

Before adopting herbal treatments into a treatment plan, contact a healthcare expert who can provide advice based on scientific evidence and your specific health requirements. Healthcare specialists may assist in assessing possible dangers, interactions, and advantages associated with individual herbs, ensuring that they are used in combination with conventional cancer therapy rather than as a replacement.

Consult With A Healthcare Provider

Consulting with a healthcare expert is an important step in determining nutritional assistance and supplements for bone cancer patients. Oncologists, certified dietitians, and integrative medicine experts may give personalized counsel based on individual requirements and treatment regimens.

During consultations, patients should share their dietary objectives, concerns, and any symptoms or side effects they are experiencing. Healthcare experts may provide suggestions for dietary changes, supplements, and lifestyle changes to improve general health and well-being during the cancer journey.

By working with a healthcare team and remaining knowledgeable about nutritional support alternatives, bone cancer patients may empower themselves to make informed decisions that promote their best health and treatment results. Regular communication and continuing monitoring may assist ensure that nutritional demands are satisfied successfully and safely during the treatment process and beyond.

CHAPTER TEN

Long-Term Nutrition And Survival

Transitioning To Post-Treatment Nutrition

Transitioning to post-treatment nutrition is a critical step in the path of bone cancer survivors. It's time to change our emphasis from fighting cancer to restoring health and energy. This shift requires cautious food choices to aid in healing and enhance general well-being.

During therapy, the body experiences tremendous stress, which often results in changes in appetite, taste preferences, and nutritional absorption. As treatment ends, survivors may endure a range of physical and mental changes as they adapt to life after cancer.

It is critical to approach a post-treatment diet with care, knowledge, and a focus on supporting the body to promote healing.

Transitioning to post-treatment nutrition includes progressively reintroducing items that were limited during treatment owing to dietary limitations or adverse effects. This technique helps survivors regain their love of eating while still meeting their nutritional requirements for healing and restoring strength. Consult with healthcare specialists or qualified dietitians to develop a personalized nutrition plan based on your specific requirements and interests.

Monitoring Bone Health

Monitoring bone health is critical for bone cancer survivors because some medications and the disease itself may affect bone density and strength. Maintaining good bone health is critical for avoiding fractures, lowering the risk of osteoporosis, and increasing general mobility and quality of life.

Regular bone density scans, also known as dual-energy X-ray absorptiometry (DEXA) scans, are usually suggested for bone cancer survivors to check bone density and detect symptoms of bone loss or weakening. Based on the findings of these scans, healthcare experts may prescribe lifestyle changes, dietary adjustments, or drugs to improve bone health.

In addition to DEXA scans, bone cancer survivors should do weight-bearing activities in their daily regimen to strengthen bones and improve balance and coordination. Walking, dancing, and weightlifting may all help to maintain bone density and lower the risk of fractures.

Regular Check-Ups And Screenings

Bone cancer survivors need regular check-ups and screenings as part of their survival treatment. These sessions let healthcare experts check for symptoms of cancer recurrence, assess treatment efficacy, and manage any remaining side effects or health issues.

During check-ups, healthcare doctors may conduct physical examinations, request blood tests, or propose imaging investigations to evaluate general health and discover any issues or anomalies. Survivors should talk freely with their healthcare provider about any symptoms or changes they are experiencing to get a quick assessment and help.

In addition to regular check-ups, survivors may be screened for additional health issues that may occur as a consequence of cancer treatment or lifestyle choices. These screenings may include testing for heart health, thyroid function, or metabolic problems, depending on the individual's risk factors and medical history.

Mental And Emotional Wellbeing

Supporting mental and emotional well-being is an important aspect of bone cancer survival therapy. A cancer diagnosis and treatment may have a profound emotional impact, and many survivors may feel anxiety, sadness, or post-traumatic stress as they adjust to life after cancer.

Survivors must prioritize self-care and seek help from healthcare providers, mental health specialists, and support groups to address any emotional issues that may arise. Mindfulness, relaxation exercises, and cognitive-behavioral therapy are among the techniques that might help survivors manage stress and enhance their coping abilities.

In addition to professional help, engaging with other survivors via support groups or online forums may give important peer support and validation. Sharing experiences, worries, and accomplishments with others who have been through a similar journey may help survivors feel more connected and empowered.

Resources And Assistance For Survivors

Accessing information and support services may significantly improve the survivorship experience for bone cancer patients. There are several tools available to help survivors navigate life after cancer, including educational materials, financial aid programs, and peer support networks.

Healthcare institutions often provide survivorship programs or clinics that provide extensive support services targeted to the requirements of cancer survivors. These programs may include dietary counseling, fitness courses, psychological support, and aid in managing long-term medical adverse effects.

In addition to local services, several national and worldwide organizations exist to help cancer survivors and their families. These organizations provide a plethora of information, advocacy, and community outreach programs to help survivors empower themselves and enhance their quality of life.

By using these resources and support networks, bone cancer survivors may get the skills, knowledge, and encouragement they need to flourish beyond illness and enjoy a happy life after treatment.

CONCLUSION

Finally, diet is critical for treating bone cancer and improving treatment results. A well-balanced diet high in key nutrients including protein, vitamins, minerals, and antioxidants may improve general health and well-being, stimulate the immune system, and assist in recovery. Adequate calorie intake is essential for avoiding malnutrition and maintaining strength throughout therapy.

Specific dietary factors, such as boosting calcium and vitamin D consumption, may aid in bone health and prevent bone loss caused by cancer therapies such as chemotherapy and radiation. Furthermore, staying hydrated and eating easy-to-digest meals may help control frequent side effects including nausea, vomiting, and lack of appetite.

While diet cannot cure bone cancer, it can help the body tolerate therapy, minimize side effects, and preserve the quality of life. As a result, persons with bone cancer must collaborate closely with a healthcare team, including a certified dietitian or nutritionist, to design a personalized nutrition plan based on their unique requirements and treatment objectives. Individuals who prioritize diet alongside medical therapy may improve their overall health and well-being during their cancer experience.

THE END

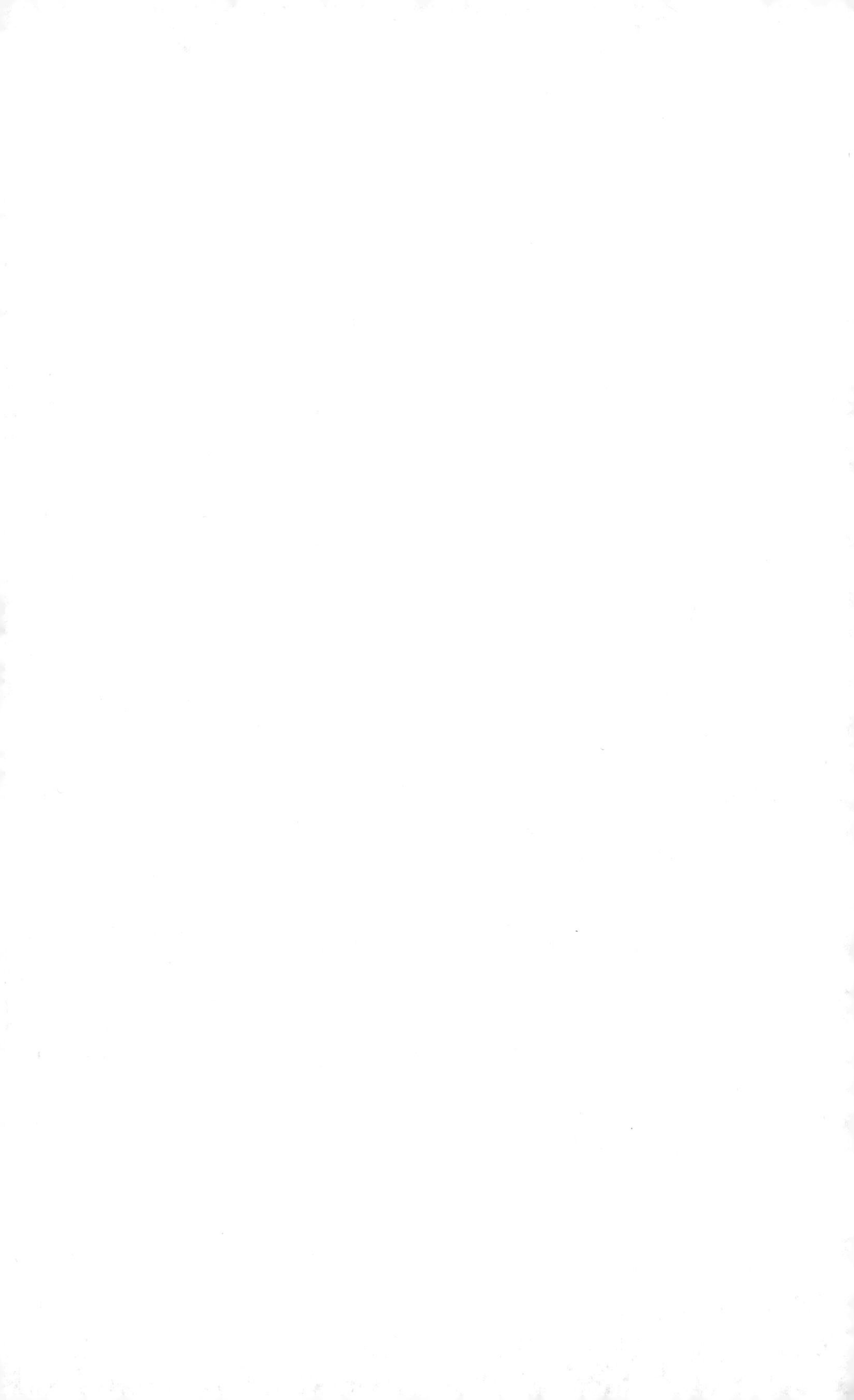

www.ingramcontent.com/pod-product-compliance
Lightning Source LLC
Chambersburg PA
CBHW050822250726
48653CB00006B/2370